Table of Contents

INTRODUCTION

More than 24 million Americans have an autoimmune disease. Scientists have identified over 80 of these conditions. An autoimmune disease is a malfunction of the immune system, wherein the immune system attacks the body. These diseases can affect many different systems of the body, and can become life-threatening if they are not treated properly. Genetics and the environment are likely risk factors for the development of an autoimmune disease.

Most of these conditions have no current cure, and sometimes, lifelong treatment is required. For those looking for additional ways to help cope with their symptoms, the AIP (autoimmune) diet may help. The Autoimmune Protocol Diet (AIP Diet) is an elimination diet that replaces food that increases the gut's permeability with nutrient-dense foods intended to help strengthen the gut and reduce symptoms associated with autoimmune disease.

It's been reported that people who follow the AIP Diet report better health and fewer symptoms of autoimmune disorders, like fatigue and pain in their joints or gut. Although the results of this diet have been promising, the research is limited. The Autoimmune Protocol Diet is an anti-inflammatory diet, and it's also an elimination diet. Elimination diets involve removing foods that you suspect your body doesn't tolerate well.

The foods are later reintroduced, one at a time, while documenting positive or adverse reactions to determine food sensitivies. In the AIP Diet, unhealthy foods are replaced with nutrient-dense, healing foods that promote gut health, reduce inflammation, and aid other symptoms of autoimmune diseases.

Certain research suggests that, in susceptible individuals, damage to the gut barrier can lead to increased intestinal permeability, otherwise known as a "leaky gut," which may contribute to the development of certain autoimmune diseases. Although experts believe that a leaky gut may be a plausible explanation for the inflammation experienced by people with autoimmune disorders, current research makes it impossible to confirm a causal relationship between the two.

The Autoimmune Protocol (AIP) Diet strives to reduce symptoms such as inflammation and pain experienced by those with autoimmune disorders by healing their leaky gut through the removal of potentially problematic ingredients from their diet. Continue reading for a comprehensive overview of the Autoimmune Protocol Diet detailing the AIP Diet and how it works.

A GUIDE TO THE AIP DIET FOR BEGINNERS

Key Takeaways:

- ✓ The autoimmune protocol diet — also called the autoimmune Paleo diet — eliminates a wide variety of foods linked with triggering inflammation for those with autoimmunity.

- ✓ The restrictive nature of the AIP diet means it shouldn't be your first choice in dealing with autoimmune symptoms.

- ✓ It makes sense to try a standard Paleo or reduced-carb (low FODMAP) regimen first, only moving onto AIP if these don't produce good enough symptom improvement.

- ✓ As well as gluten, AIP eliminates dairy, legumes, grains, nightshade vegetables (e.g. tomatoes, peppers, and potatoes), nuts, seeds, eggs, and seed-derived spices.

✓ Some studies have shown the AIP diet can improve the symptoms of Hashimoto's thyroiditis, IBD, and other autoimmune conditions.

✓ After the initial elimination phase of the AIP diet, it's important to reintroduce foods one by one, watching out for symptoms.

✓ Over time you can use what you've learned about your food sensitivities to create a maintenance diet that works for you.

Being diagnosed with an autoimmune disease like Hashimoto's thyroiditis or inflammatory bowel disease, or experiencing autoimmune symptoms such as joint pain, brain fog, fatigue, and gut pain can be distressing. But it's good to know that various types of elimination diets, including the autoimmune protocol (AIP) diet for more intractable cases, may reduce your symptoms and improve your quality of life.

However, It's important to understand that, in spite of the name, an autoimmune protocol diet is not necessary for everyone who has an autoimmune disease. You'd be better off trying less restrictive diets first and only moving onto the AIP if these don't work for you (or this diet has been specifically recommended for you). The AIP diet can be a little daunting, but over time you'll generally find a version of it that works for you.

Once you know the basics of an AIP diet for beginners (which we'll go through in this article), the rest is generally personalizing the diet to achieve the best results for your specific symptoms. Before getting into the details, here's a quick overview.

How Diet Can Help Autoimmune Conditions

Autoimmune conditions include:

- ✓ Hashimoto's thyroiditis
- ✓ Lupus

- ✓ Rheumatoid arthritis
- ✓ Multiple sclerosis
- ✓ Graves' disease
- ✓ Addison's disease
- ✓ Celiac disease

Excessive inflammation underlies many autoimmune conditions, which is where changes to your diet can help. By removing potentially inflammatory foods that may aggravate your symptoms, you can achieve some symptom relief. Identifying your worst trigger foods and then continuing to avoid them can help to maintain your autoimmune symptoms at a lower level. Here are some general principles for an elimination and reintroduction approach:

- ✓ Start with the least restrictive diet framework possible.
- ✓ Follow your new diet for two to three weeks and observe symptoms.

- ✓ If symptoms improve, gradually reintroduce healthy foods while monitoring how you feel.
- ✓ If symptoms don't resolve, try a more specialized diet.

In my clinical experience, it's usually best to start with a lighter intervention first. For many people with autoimmune illnesses, a Paleo diet, which focuses on unprocessed whole foods close to the pattern humans were eating in Paleolithic times, is sufficiently anti-inflammatory to ease symptoms. For others, the low FODMAP diet, which removes the fermentable carbohydrates that trigger some gut bacteria to produce a lot of gas, is helpful.

However, if neither of these diets works well, or if you experience just limited success with a standard Paleo diet, the more advanced AIP may be the best diet for you, at least in the short term.

There are three parts to any elimination diet: the elimination phase, the reintroduction phase and the maintenance phase. Here's how to work the AIP diet into your daily life for the best results.

Elimination Phase

You'll likely already be gluten-free and dairy-free if you are eating Paleo. If this or a carb reduction (low FODMAP) diet hasn't worked to resolve your autoimmune symptoms, the initial elimination phase of the AIP diet is more likely to have a symptom-easing effect because it cuts out a much wider range of foods, including eggs, grains, legumes, nuts and seeds, added sweeteners, alcohol, nightshade veggies, and processed foods.

To get started on the elimination phase of AIP, check the guide below for a list of foods to eat or avoid). If you don't see any symptom improvement after two to three weeks, it's likely that your symptoms aren't related to the foods you eliminated on the AIP diet. If you do notice improvement, continue the elimination phase until your symptomatic improvements plateau.

Reintroductions

Once you have reached a plateau, it's time to begin reintroductions. Reintroduce one food at a time, and watch for any change in symptoms. It's most practical to start your reintroductions with the foods you miss most. Use a food diary to help you. If you have a symptom flare after reintroducing a food, that food may need to stay out of your diet for a while longer. If you don't notice any symptoms, you can safely include it in your diet again.

If you do notice a symptom flare when reintroducing a particular food, try not to get discouraged! This doesn't necessarily mean you'll need to avoid the food forever. Your body may just need a bit more time to heal. Try reintroducing the food again after a few more weeks, or whenever you feel most comfortable.

Maintenance Phase

Once you've reintroduced all the foods you want to test, use what you learned to create a custom diet plan that minimizes your symptoms while you focus on improving your gut health and other treatments.

Tips for Success

- ✓ Making any diet change can feel overwhelming and challenging at first, so to make the AIP diet for beginners easier, try these few tips:
- ✓ Find a few basic recipes that sound good and use them to develop a simple meal plan. Once you're comfortable with your dietary changes and know which foods trigger your symptoms, research new recipes to expand your menu options.

✓ Stock your pantry with ingredients you need for your basic meal plan, and remove all off-AIP plan foods. Make a few big batches of your simple starter recipes and load up your freezer.

✓ Be as strict as possible about the diet during the first two to three weeks. This will help you feel better faster and give you better results during your food reintroductions.

Research on AIP and Autoimmunity

Overall, studies of the AIP diet for autoimmune disease are still in short supply. But what we have adds credence to the hypothesis that it seems to help some people with autoimmune conditions.

Consider these study results:

✓ An 11-week AIP diet for patients with active inflammatory bowel disease (IBD) improved their quality of life.

- ✓ Women with Hashimoto's thyroiditis improved their quality of life and symptoms by using the AIP diet for 10 weeks. After following the AIP diet for Hashimoto's, inflammation in these women decreased by an impressive 29%.
- ✓ Inflammatory bowel disease patients who used the autoimmune protocol diet saw significantly improved IBD scores. Follow-up endoscopies after 11 weeks on the diet showed signs of mucosal healing in some patients.

AIP and Autoantibodies

Autoantibodies (misguided, or pathogenic, antibodies produced in response to your body's own proteins), are the hallmark of many autoimmune ailments. Higher levels of autoantibodies tend to correlate with a more significant autoimmune disease and greater clinical symptoms When levels of these fall, it tends to imply improvement in a patient's autoimmune condition.

To date, no studies have shown that the AIP diet, specifically, reduces autoantibodies. However, a small-scale systematic review (6 case studies and 2 clinical trials) found the standard Paleo diet reduced thyroid antibodies and normalized thyroid hormones in Hashimoto's thyroiditis and Graves' disease. More research is needed, but this is an encouraging finding.

It implies that an anti-inflammatory diet in general, and potentially the AIP diet more specifically, may target the underlying causes of autoimmunity.

Other Nutrient-Rich Diets and Autoimmunity

A few additional studies of interventions similar to the AIP diet have also found encouraging improvements for people with autoimmune illnesses. For example, the Wahls Paleo diet, which is similar to the AIP diet (i.e. a Paleo diet modified to reduce autoimmunity), improved fatigue, disability, and quality of life in those with relapsing-remitting multiple sclerosis according to one meta-analysis.

MS patients following the Wahls diet also experienced better mental health with reduced depression and anxiety. In a nutshell, there's enough inferential evidence to warrant trying the AIP diet for autoimmune conditions if you haven't seen any symptom relief from a less-restrictive diet like the Paleo diet.

Downside of an AIP Diet

While the AIP diet can offer immediate relief for more complicated autoimmune cases, I am concerned the initial elimination stage can potentially result in nutrient deficiencies if you carry it on too long. Ultimately this may worsen the underlying issues that created the autoimmunity in the first place. This is why I always recommend that you try a more moderate version of a paleo diet first.

If you do progress to the AIP diet, it's vital you move on to the reintroduction and maintenance phases as soon as you are able. It might be worth having some professional help with these later stages of the AIP diet — you can reach out to us at the Ruscio Institute if you think this would benefit you.

Understanding Autoimmune Disease

Autoimmune disease happens because your immune system mistakenly attacks your own tissues. Depending on which part of your body is being attacked, you may experience a wide range of symptoms, from fatigue to skin rashes, bloating and other gut problems, thyroid health issues, and chronic pain. Autoimmune disorders affect approximately 16% of Americans and appear to be increasing in prevalence.

Women account for 78% of autoimmune disease patients. Quality of life can be low for autoimmune patients whose disease isn't under control. Some of the most common autoimmune diseases are:

- ✓ Inflammatory bowel diseases, like Crohn's disease and celiac disease
- ✓ The thyroid disorders Hashimoto's thyroiditis and Graves' disease
- ✓ Rheumatoid arthritis
- ✓ Lupus (systemic lupus erythematosus or SLE)
- ✓ Psoriasis
- ✓ Multiple sclerosis (MS)
- ✓ Type 1 diabetes
- ✓ Swollen glands or lymph nodes

The Gut-Autoimmune Link

Your genes and stress level are two factors that can affect your chances of developing an autoimmune condition. However, disruptions in gut microbiota are also now thought to play a major role. Out-of-balance gut bacteria can increase intestinal permeability, which causes a cascade of inflammation and an overzealous immune response. Increased intestinal permeability (a leaky gut) is thought to be particularly closely related to the development of autoimmune disease.

When you remove inflammatory foods, as happens in the AIP and other elimination diets, inflammation decreases, which may help to heal your gut lining and calm your overactive immune response. In addition to dietary changes, you can give yourself a helping hand by taking a well-formulated probiotic supplement. Probiotics have been shown to:

- ✓ Help reduce intestinal permeability.
- ✓ Promote a healthy immune response in your gut.
- ✓ Probiotics are natural helpers for autoimmune patients.

The AIP Diet is Worth a Try

If you have an autoimmune disease and haven't seen any symptom relief from a basic elimination diet like the Paleo diet, the autoimmune protocol diet is a worthwhile option. It's been shown to reduce symptoms and improve quality of life for inflammatory bowel disease and autoimmune thyroid disease patients. Try the AIP diet for beginners with confidence by keeping things simple, creating a simplified meal plan, and preparing your pantry.

Only stick with the diet after the first several weeks if you're seeing symptom improvement.

AIP FOOD LIST: WHAT YOU SHOULD BE EATING

Popular among anti-inflammatory diets and a close relative of the paleo diet, an AIP diet is a relatively new lifestyle approach. But what exactly does it entail and which foods are AIP approved?

What You Need to Know About an Autoimmune Protocol Diet

An AIP diet or autoimmune protocol diet is believed by some, to support gut health and reduce inflammation associated with autoimmune diseases like crohn's disease and rheumatoid arthritis. However, the link between metabolism and the immune system is not well understood and scientists are only beginning to tap into the relationship between food and inflammation.

In other words, this style of eating is not heavily rooted in science and may not offer any advantages over a basic healthy diet. And if you have an autoimmune condition, you are likely much better off following medical advice from a trained physician or dietitian. Regardless, there likely isn't any harm to trying AIP either as long as you focus on good nutrition and feeding your body the food it needs to thrive.

How to Start an AIP Diet

If you are interested in trying an AIP eating plan, here's some tips to go about it in a healthy way.

1. Use portion control

Regardless of what type of diet or lifestyle you choose to follow, calorie control is the only known, proven approach to weight management. Meaning, if you are looking to lose weight or even maintain your weight on AIP, portion control is essential. Start by figuring out how many calories you need each day and then build your AIP approved menu to match!

2. Balance Your Nutrition

The quality of your calories matter when it comes to your health - this means finding the right balance of macronutrients and micronutrients with your meals. Getting enough protein, carbs, and healthy fats along with essential vitamins and minerals can support improved mood, energy levels, and help manage diet related chronic illness.

3. Be Flexible

AIP is technically an elimination diet - meaning you cut out specific foods for a certain time period and then gradually add them back in, one by one. This method allows you to determine if any specific foods are causing discomfort or noticeable symptoms so that you can avoid them for the foreseeable future. Follow a menu based on the suggested food lists below for two to three weeks and then slowly start adding these foods back in, paying close attention to how your body feels is key.

What Foods Should You Initially Avoid on an AIP Diet?

Backers of the AIP diet believe that heavily processed, modern foods like refined grains, dairy, sugar, and alcohol can lead to increased inflammation and intestinal permeability resulting in something referred to as "leaky gut". But this is not a defined medical condition and not proven with research. AIP also restricts some nutritious foods that some believe may irritate your gut including nightshades, nuts, seeds, legumes, and eggs.

But, again, there is not any research to suggest that these foods negatively impact your health. In addition to nearly all processed foods, the recommended foods to restrict on AIP include:

- ✓ Alcohol
- ✓ Chlorella
- ✓ Coffee
- ✓ Dairy

- ✓ Eggs
- ✓ Eggplant
- ✓ Goji berries
- ✓ Grains
- ✓ Legumes
- ✓ Nuts
- ✓ Peppers
- ✓ Potatoes (except sweet potatoes and yams)
- ✓ Seeds
- ✓ Seed oils: canola oil, sesame oil, sunflower oil, etc.
- ✓ Spirulina
- ✓ Sugars
- ✓ Tomatoes

Adding These Foods Back In

Because AIP is an elimination diet, you don't need to avoid these foods forever. After a few weeks, start to add back in your favorite options and see if it makes a difference to how you are feeling.

Just because a food "fits" into the AIP criteria does not mean you can eat as much as you want. Calorie control is still crucial to weight management. Additionally, your overall nutrition intake has a major impact on your long term health and wellbeing - likely more so than following an AIP diet in the first place. To ensure you get the most nutrition while sticking to your AIP diet list, here are the best foods to add to you AIP meal plan.

Meat and Fish

Grass-fed, organic proteins and sustainably caught fish are a great way to get lean protein and nutrition into your diet. Eating seafood, especially fatty fish, is one of the best ways to get important omega-3 fatty acids linked to improved heart health, brain health, and potentially reduced inflammation. In addition, diets high in protein are associated with many positive health weight loss benefits including supporting lean muscle mass, and reduced cravings and hunger.

To get some of these potential benefits, aim to get roughly 20% to 30% of your daily calories from lean protein each day. Here are some of the best sources of protein to stock up on:

- ✓ Anchovies
- ✓ Antelope
- ✓ Bison
- ✓ Cod
- ✓ Chicken
- ✓ Crab
- ✓ Clams
- ✓ Duck
- ✓ Elk
- ✓ Goat
- ✓ Grass-fed beef and steak
- ✓ Herring
- ✓ Ostrich
- ✓ Pork

- ✓ Lamb
- ✓ Lobster
- ✓ Mackerel
- ✓ Mussels
- ✓ Oysters
- ✓ Salmon
- ✓ Sardines
- ✓ Scallops
- ✓ Shrimp
- ✓ Tilapia
- ✓ Tuna
- ✓ Turkey
- ✓ Venison

Vegetables for AIP foods list

Nearly all veggies are AIP approved with the exception of nightshades (noted above). Vegetables, especially non-starchy veggies, are nutrient dense superfoods - with many high in essential micronutrients and low in calories. Plus, research suggests that a balanced diet high in veggies can promote improved health and may play a role reducing inflammation.

Stack your plate with high amounts of the following veggies:

- ✓ Acorn squash
- ✓ Artichokes
- ✓ Asparagus
- ✓ Avocado
- ✓ Beets
- ✓ Bok Choy
- ✓ Broccoli
- ✓ Brussels sprouts
- ✓ Cabbage
- ✓ Carrots
- ✓ Cassava
- ✓ Cauliflower
- ✓ Celery
- ✓ Chicory
- ✓ Cucumber
- ✓ Fennel

- ✓ Fresh Herbs: basil, cilantro, oregano, parsley, thyme, etc.
- ✓ Green onions/scallions
- ✓ Jicama
- ✓ Kohlrabi
- ✓ Leafy greens: arugula, collards, endive, dandelion, kale, lettuce, mustard greens, romaine, spinach, Swiss chard, turnip greens, watercress, etc.
- ✓ Leeks
- ✓ Mushrooms
- ✓ Okra
- ✓ Onions
- ✓ Parsley
- ✓ Parsnips
- ✓ Pumpkin
- ✓ Radicchio
- ✓ Radish
- ✓ Rutabaga
- ✓ Seaweed
- ✓ Summer squash

- ✓ Sweet Potato

- ✓ Taro

- ✓ Turnips

- ✓ Watercress

- ✓ Winter Squash

- ✓ Yams

- ✓ Zucchini

AIP fruits

While higher in natural sugars than veggies, fruits are also a good source of nutrition and fiber for good health.

AIP approved fruits include:

- ✓ Apples

- ✓ Apricots

- ✓ Bananas

- ✓ Blackberries

- ✓ Blueberries

- ✓ Cantaloupe

- ✓ Cherries

✓ Coconut

✓ Cranberries

✓ Dates

✓ Figs

✓ Grapefruit

✓ Grapes

✓ Guava

✓ Melon

✓ Kiwi

✓ Lemon

✓ Lime

✓ Lychee

✓ Mandarins

✓ Mango

✓ Nectarines

✓ Oranges

✓ Olives

✓ Papaya

✓ Passion Fruit

✓ Peaches

✓ Pears

✓ Persimmons

✓ Pineapple

✓ Plums

✓ Pomegranates

✓ Raspberries

✓ Rhubarb

✓ Star Fruit

✓ Strawberries

✓ Tangerines

✓ Watermelon

Butter and Oils

Seed oils and heavily processed fats and oils are restricted with AIP, but there are still many heart healthy sources of fat you can enjoy, including:

✓ Avocado oil

✓ Coconut oil

✓ Olive oil

AIP Fermented Foods

Because AIP is rooted in prompting better gut health, fermented foods are commonly encouraged. As a source of natural probiotics, some studies imply that fermented foods can support improved general health and your immune function. But, while the research surrounding fermented foods and gut microbiota is fascinating, much more research is needed to determine how effective these foods truly are.

Popular fermented health foods include:

- ✓ Coconut milk kefir and yogurt
- ✓ Kombucha
- ✓ Pickled veggies
- ✓ Sauerkraut
- ✓ White kimchi

Other Specialty Foods

Other specialty foods that commonly have gut health claims (most of which are not proven with research) and are considered AIP friendly include:

- ✓ Bone broth
- ✓ Collagen
- ✓ Vinegar.

AIP DIET FOR BEGINNERS: WHAT TO KNOW ABOUT THE AIP DIET

Key Takeaways:

- ✓ Inflammation is your body's attempt at healing after being harmed or exposed to viruses, bacteria, illnesses, or other stressors.

- ✓ The autoimmune protocol diet eliminates trigger foods and may decrease inflammation in the gut.

- ✓ A registered dietitian can help you follow the autoimmune diet and manage your symptoms.

- ✓ Living with chronic inflammation can be overwhelming and painful. Confusion about what to eat and what to avoid can add even more stress to your day.

But here is some good news: following the Autoimmune Protocol Diet (or the AIP diet plan) could relieve inflammation in the digestive tract and may help you feel better. There are three components of the AIP diet. Eliminate food triggers that are gut-irritating, maintain these changes for 30-90 days, and end the protocol by reintroducing foods into your diet.

Meaning of Autoimmune

Your immune system includes your lymphatic system and white blood cells. They're constantly screening for harmful germs, bacteria, or viruses that could make you sick. Your white blood cells are signaled if a threat is identified. Activating your white blood cells is a normal inflammatory response that keeps you healthy. Once the germ or pathogen is destroyed, the inflammation will subside.

Autoimmune disorders are when your immune system targets pathogens and healthy organs and tissues in the body. It can lead to a chronic state of inflammation and significantly decrease quality of life. A few side effects of long-term inflammation include constant fatigue, swelling, pain all over the body, and skin changes.

Examples of Autoimmune Diseases

This is a shortened list of common diagnoses:

- ✓ Type 1 Diabetes.
- ✓ Lupus.
- ✓ Rheumatoid Arthritis.
- ✓ Thyroid diseases, including Graves disease, resulting in an overactive thyroid (hyperthyroidism). Or Hashimoto's, which leads to an underactive thyroid (hypothyroidism).
- ✓ Psoriasis.

There are no cures for these conditions but they can be managed through evidence-based practices. These include Tdietary strategies (the AIP diet may work for some people), regular physical activity, and medications.

Meaning of AIP Diet

The Autoimmune Protocol (AIP) is sometimes also called the Autoimmune Paleolithic Diet. It was developed to reduce inflammation by eliminating trigger foods which contain organic compounds and proteins that may worsen digestive inflammatory responses. The AIP diet is not the same as the low FODMAP diet, which helps people reduce symptoms linked to carbohydrate intake.

By following the AIP diet plan and eliminating these foods, the inflammatory response decreases. A break in inflammation offers the body a chance to recover, and the lining of the gut wall can heal. We know this restrictive diet plan is not suitable for everyone. It could help people who suffer from chronic inflammation related to an autoimmune condition.

The AIP diet is a stricter version of the Paleolithic diet. It doesn't permit anything processed or ultra-processed (UPF), including cookies, chips, crackers, candy, breakfast cereals, etc. Instead, this diet includes various vegetables, fruits, lean protein sources including seafood, and some plant-based milks. There are known adverse health effects associated with a high intake of UPFs.

Health risks include unwanted weight gain, heart disease, and different forms of cancer, specifically colon cancer. UPFs are notoriously high in excess refined sugars, fats, and salt. Consuming large amounts of these ingredients may contribute to high levels of inflammation. For these reasons, UPFs are not recommended in the AIP diet plan.

Here are examples of other foods that are not AIP-compatible:

- ✓ Nightshade vegetables: Examples include all tomato varieties, eggplant, potatoes, and peppers (including sweet bell peppers and spicy chilis).

✓ Nuts and seeds: Only eliminate nuts, nut butter, and seeds from the diet if they worsen your symptoms. Most people don't need to restrict 100% of these foods.

✓ All grains.

✓ Legumes and beans.

✓ Coffee and Alcohol.

✓ Eggs.

✓ Refined sugars, including white sugar, brown sugar, and high fructose corn syrup.

✓ Animal-based dairy products.

Keep in mind that everybody's health and digestion are unique. This list is just a guideline. As you move through the AIP diet plan, you'll establish a version that best suits your needs. If you want support, consider booking an online appointment with a Nourish dietitian specializing in inflammation.

The AIP Diet Plan Has Three Phases:

- ✓ Elimination Phase: four to six weeks of eliminating common trigger foods that may increase your body's inflammatory response. This phase of the diet is temporary.

- ✓ Maintenance Phase: maintain the elimination diet for 30-90 days. Ensure you have included nutrient dense foods in your diet. If your symptoms have not resolved after 90 days, you may need to explore other options with your healthcare team.

- ✓ Reintroduction Phase: if you feel better, try reintroducing foods back into your diet. Approach this phase as scientifically as possible. Write a list of foods you want to bring back into your diet and reintroduce them one at a time. Allow seven days between each food.

Inflammatory Bowel Disease

Inflammatory bowel disease (IBD) includes Crohn's disease and Ulcerative Colitis. People can manage both conditions through diet, but painful flare-ups can occur. During a flare-up, the intestinal walls become inflamed, and the digestive tract is sensitive to different foods and beverages. These acute events may lead to fatigue, fever, diarrhea, blood in the stool, and a decreased appetite.

A research study from 2017 observed 15 participants who followed the AIP diet for approximately three weeks. At 11 weeks, the participants completed an endoscopy (an imaging test with a scope), and visible inflammation along the gut walls had decreased. People who suffer from IBD conditions may benefit from the AIP diet plan.

Hashimotos

Hashimotos is an autoimmune disorder that targets and destroys thyroid cells. It results in the underproduction of thyroid hormone (clinically known as hypothyroidism). Most people will rely on medication to manage their thyroid levels. A study from 2019 looked at the role of the AIP diet in people diagnosed with Hashimotos. Participants had blood drawn at the start and end of the study.

Researcher's were checking thyroid and c-reactive protein levels. High levels of c-protein can be an indication of inflammation. After ten weeks, the TSH levels in participants were the same, but the c-protein had decreased. The sample size of this study is small and more research with a larger population would strengthen the findings. The AIP diet plan may help people who have been diagnosed with Hashimotos.

Leaky Gut

Leaky gut is not an official diagnosis in western medicine, but it's a trending topic in the nutrition world. The current definition of a leaky gut is the increased permeability (or passability) of intestinal walls. There is an increased risk of germs and bacteria passing into the surrounding tissues of the gut. Unwanted germs and bacteria contribute to inflammation and may cause significant pain.

Studies have confirmed that other autoimmune conditions, such as Crohn's, have permeable intestinal walls, contributing to poor gut health and uncomfortable symptoms. The AIP diet plan may improve the leaky gut by decreasing the inflammatory response to foods. Less stress on the gut will give it a chance to heal and recover.

How Does Diet Help Autoimmune Conditions?

A diet rich in antioxidants may decrease symptoms of inflammation associated with autoimmune conditions. Antioxidant rich foods include fruits and vegetables, fiber-rich grains, beans, and unsaturated fats. The nutrients in these foods neutralize harmful free radicals, which are compounds that could worsen inflammation if levels become too high.

Additionally, research has demonstrated that people with autoimmune conditions who eat anti-inflammatory diets have lower levels of mortality.

A Shopping List for the AIP Diet

Below are recommendations for an AIP-friendly grocery list.

- ✓ Lean ground proteins including turkey, chicken, and beef.
- ✓ Fish rich in omega-3 fatty acids such as salmon and trout. Other fish you can buy include cod, haddock, tilapia, and tuna.
- ✓ Seafood, including shrimp and scallops.

✓ Most vegetables are AIP-compliant except for nightshade options. Include broccoli, cabbage, mushrooms, turnips, zucchini, garlic, brussel sprouts, and onion.

✓ Starchy vegetables such as sweet potatoes, yams, and squashes.

✓ Most fresh fruits, including berries, apples, oranges, nectarines, pomegranates, and bananas.

✓ Coconut milk.

✓ Honey.

✓ Olive oil, avocado oil.

Sample AIP Meal Plan

Here's an example of a three-day AIP diet plan you can try at home.

Day 1

Breakfast: Sweet potato "toast" (a slice of roasted sweet potato) topped with mashed avocado and spices, such as turmeric and ground cumin.

Lunch: Baked tuna cakes served over fresh spinach and drizzled with olive oil and balsamic vinegar.

Dinner: One-pan chicken with rosemary, parsnips, garlic, and fresh thyme. Glaze the dish with avocado oil, salt, cinnamon, and one tablespoon of maple syrup.

Day 2

Breakfast: Cassava flour pancakes topped with mixed berries.

Lunch: Nori fish wraps with avocado and pickled vegetables.

Dinner: Grass-fed steak with a green salad and sauteed mushrooms and squash on the side.

Day 3

Breakfast: Toast large coconut flakes to create a cold cereal texture and top with fresh fruits and coconut milk.

Lunch: Chicken lettuce wraps with homemade AIP-friendly caesar dressing and sliced avocado.

Dinner: Mediterranean-style shrimp cooked on a pan with olive oil, minced garlic, oregano, and basil. Served with baked zucchini, carrots, and sweet potatoes.

Are There Any Risks of the AIP Diet Plan?

The AIP diet plan can result in low fiber intake because it eliminates whole grains, legumes, several vegetables, nuts, and seeds, which are all high sources of fiber. Low fiber intake is linked to several diseases, including cancer, heart disease, type two diabetes, constipation, and diverticular disease.

Minimum Daily Fiber Recommendations

Women (ages 19-30): 28g

Women (ages 31-50): 25g

Women (ages 51+): 22g

Men (ages 19-30): 34g

Men (ages 31-50): 31g

Men (ages 51+): 28g

In the most recent USDA Dietary Guidelines it was noted that more than 90% of women and 97% of men are not meeting recommended dietary fiber goals. These numbers are staggeringly high. You should create a robust AIP diet plan that prioritizes high-fiber vegetables and fruits to help you satisfy your fiber requirements. These include avocados, berries, broccoli, cabbages, and other cruciferous vegetables.

The Fear of Moving Forward

People who have suffered from chronic inflammation may find relief after starting the AIP diet plan. Understandably, they may be afraid to move out of the elimination phase, fearing the pain and discomfort will return. It is essential to move on to the reintroduction phase because a sustainable diet needs variety. If you feel stuck or fearful, reach out to a friend or, even better, a trained dietitian. They can offer actionable steps to move forwards while still maintaining your progress.

Tips for Success:

- ✓ Small, consistent nutrition changes are gentler on your digestive system and easier to follow. Here are other tips you can follow:
- ✓ Focus on one meal at a time.
- ✓ Work with an expert, such as a dietitian specializing in inflammation.
- ✓ Make simple recipes that are easy to follow.
- ✓ Document your symptoms to track any changes.
- ✓ Batch cook meals or components to prepare for the week ahead.
- ✓ Prepare AIP-friendly snacks to satisfy unexpected hunger pangs.

✓ Practice mindfulness at meals.

✓ Book an appointment with a dietitian

Takeaway

AIP is an elimination diet designed to help you identify food-triggered irritations. People who suffer from autoimmune conditions or leaky gut are the best candidates to try the AIP diet plan. Remember that the diet has three phases and is a long-term commitment. People with an advanced understanding of nutrition can start the diet independently.

However, beginners with no nutrition education should ask for help to make safe nutrition choices. Avoid staying in the elimination phase for too long because it can expose you to nutritional deficiencies. The AIP diet plan can be low in fiber, and a low fiber intake can worsen your long-term health. Limit your risk by prioritizing fiber-rich foods at all meals, starting with breakfast.

Challenge yourself to try new recipes and include as much variety in your meal plan. If you struggle with cooking daily, consider meal prepping a few dishes in advance.

How a Dietitian Can Help

The path to a healthier, happier you isn't always straightforward. Partner with autoimmune dietitians at Nourish for help achieving health and wellness through personalized nutrition counseling. Find a dietitian near you by tapping into our national telehealth network of online dietitians who accept insurance.

Food Reintroduction Process

Here's a step-by-step approach (similar to the paleo approach) on reintroducing foods avoided during the initial elimination phase of the Auto Immune Protocol Diet. Reintroduction Prep: choose one item of food to reintroduce to your diet. You will consume the selected food a couple of times per day on the day of testing and then avoid it entirely for 5-7 days after testing.

Step 1. Eat a small amount of the selected food, about one teaspoon, and then wait 15-30 minutes to see if you have any reaction.

Step 2. If you experience any negative symptoms, end the test and avoid the food immediately. If no symptoms occur, eat a slightly larger portion of the same food, about two tablespoons, and monitor how you feel for the next few hours.

Step 3. If you experience any symptoms during this time of testing, end the test and avoid the food immediately. If no symptoms occur, eat a regular portion of the same food and avoid it for 5–6 days without reintroducing any other foods.

Step 4. If you don't experience any symptoms for 5–7 days, you may begin to slowly reincorporate the tested food into your diet.

Step 5. Repeat the 4-step reintroduction process above with a new food item.

It's advised to avoid reintroducing foods under circumstances that increase inflammation because it will be more difficult to interpret test results. Circumstances that may increase inflammation include: following a poor night's sleep, during an infection, following a strenuous workout, or when feeling unusually stressed. Additionally, it's seldom recommended to reintroduce foods in a particular order to reduce the risks of extreme adverse effects.

For example, when reintroducing dairy, you may want to reintroduce products with the lowest lactose concentration first.

Foods to Avoid and Foods to Eat

The elimination phase of the AIP Diet follows strict recommendations in terms of which foods to eat or avoid. It's a good idea to create an AIP Diet meal plan and shopping list for yourself based on the foods to eat and avoid during the elimination phase.

Foods to Avoid

Foods to avoid on the AIP Diet include nuts, seeds, grains, legumes, dairy, eggs, food additives, nightshade vegetables, and processed foods—including processed vegetable oils and processed sugars. The consumption of drugs such as caffeine, alcohol, and tobacco should also be avoided.

Avoid the following Foods:

- ✓ Grains
- ✓ Alcohol
- ✓ Eggs
- ✓ Alcohol
- ✓ Coffee
- ✓ Cocoa
- ✓ Legumes such as beans, lentils, and soy

- ✓ Dairy products such as milk, cheese, and yogurt
- ✓ Nuts and seeds such as peanuts, almonds, and sesame seeds
- ✓ Nightshade vegetables such as eggplants, peppers, and tomatoes
- ✓ Processed foods
- ✓ Refined carbohydrates
- ✓ Processed and refined sugars
- ✓ Artificial sweeteners
- ✓ Refined vegetable oils, nut oils, and seed oils.
- ✓ Nightshade spices such as paprika and seed-based spices, such as coriander and cumin
- ✓ NSAID's such as Ibuprofen and aspirin
- ✓ Preservatives, thickeners, flavorings, emulsifiers, coloring, and other food additives such as guar gum.

Foods to Eat

Despite being allowed, some protocols recommend moderating intake of certain foods such as salt, saturated fats, coconut-based foods, and natural sugars such as honey, maple syrup. Additionally, some protocols recommend limiting high-glycemic fruits and vegetables.

- ✓ Animal protein such as meat, organ meat, and fish
- ✓ Animal fats such as duck lard and beef tallow
- ✓ Animal bone broth
- ✓ Fermented foods such as kombucha, kimchi, and sauerkraut
- ✓ Leafy green vegetables such as chard, spinach, and kale
- ✓ Brassicas such as brussels sprouts, cauliflower, and broccoli
- ✓ Green vegetables such as asparagus, zucchini, and cucumbers

- ✓ Root vegetables such as sweet potatoes, taro, and yams
- ✓ Minimally processed oils such as avocado oil, coconut oil, and olive oil
- ✓ Non-seed based AIP-approved herbs and spices
- ✓ Coconut flakes, coconut milk, and coconut aminos
- ✓ Natural vinegars sans added sugar, such as apple cider vinegar
- ✓ Natural starches such as arrowroot starch and tapioca starch.

25+ EAST & MOUTHWATERING AIP DIET RECIPES

Figuring out what to eat for dinner on the autoimmune protocol (AIP) diet can be stressful. If you're feeling overwhelmed or burnt out when it comes to recipe creation, we've got you covered. From one pan meals to breakfasts and soups, we've got you covered. These AIP diet recipes are easy, quick, and delicious, and of course, AIP compliant.

Remember, while following the AIP Diet you want to eliminate inflammatory foods, emphasize nutrient-dense food, and after a period of strict elimination, slowly start reintroducing them to yourself. Here is a quick reminder of what you can and cannot include in your meal planning on the AIP Diet.

What you can eat on the AIP diet: mostly fruits and vegetables, grass fed/organic meat, fish, healthy fats and oils, coconut products, and grain/nut-free starches and flours. What you can't eat on the AIP diet: nightshades, nuts, seeds, alcohol, eggs, anything artificial, cane sugar, cacao, caffeine, alcohol, gums, legumes, dairy, and grains.

25 Mouthwatering and Easy AIP Diet Recipes

1. Lemon and Asparagus Chicken Skillet

Ingredients:

- ✓ Chicken Breast
- ✓ Asparagus
- ✓ Garlic, green onion, salt and pepper
- ✓ Lemon Juice
- ✓ Chicken Broth
- ✓ Coconut Aminos
- ✓ Arrowroot Starch

AIP sheet pan recipes are some of our favorite protocol recipes. This one-pan meal comes together in under 45 minutes and offers you a light, fresh, and flavorful meal. Grab the Lemon and Asparagus Chicken Skillet recipe over at Unbound Wellness.

2. Sweet Potato Chicken Poppers

Ingredients:

- ✓ Ground Chicken
- ✓ Sweet Potato
- ✓ Coconut Flour
- ✓ Garlic Powder
- ✓ Onion Powder
- ✓ Green Onion

These poppers are AIP, gluten free, paleo free, AND egg free, all while still being so delicious that people on no diet at all will want to devour them. They're veggie packed and offer you a more mature version of those classic chicken nuggets everybody knows and loves. Grab the Sweet Potato Chicken Poppers Recipe over at Unbound Wellness.

3. Cozy Instant Pot Chili

Ingredients:

- ✓ Ground Meat
- ✓ Onion
- ✓ Garlic
- ✓ Root Veggies
- ✓ Herbs
- ✓ Spices
- ✓ Pumpkin Puree
- ✓ Bone Broth

Who doesn't love a good comforting pot of chili? You probably thought you can't eat chili on the AIP diet because you should avoid eating tomatoes and beans; however, think again! This delicious and cozy recipe is tomato and bean free. Packed with various veggies and flavors, this is sure to keep your taste buds and gut happy.

4. Tropical Chicken Salad

Ingredients:

- ✓ Chicken Breasts
- ✓ Red Lettuce
- ✓ Mango
- ✓ Red Onion
- ✓ Avocado
- ✓ Lime Juice
- ✓ Cilantro
- ✓ Plantain Chips
- ✓ Unsweetened Coconut

If you're looking for a refreshing summertime meal, look no further than this tropical chicken salad. Filled with ingredients like chicken, mango, lime, cilantro and avocado, this is going to be your new favorite meal. It's extremely delicious and only takes 8 minutes to throw together. It really doesn't get much better than this.

5. One Pan Chicken Pesto

Ingredients:

- ✓ Chicken Thighs
- ✓ Carrots
- ✓ Zucchinis
- ✓ Broccoli Florets
- ✓ Red Onion
- ✓ Sea Salt and Pepper

A great one pan dinner option that's delicious yet easy. This recipe also features a simple homemade pesto sauce you'll want to top everything with!

6. Beef and Kale Casserole

Ingredients:

- ✓ Ground Beef
- ✓ Celery
- ✓ Kale
- ✓ Nomato Sauce
- ✓ Coconut Milk

- ✓ Apple Cider Vinegar
- ✓ Tapioca Starch
- ✓ Turmeric.

7. Gluten Free Copycat Hamburger Helper

Ingredients:

- ✓ Ground Beef
- ✓ Canned Coconut Milk
- ✓ Tomato Sauce
- ✓ Onion
- ✓ Seasoning
- ✓ Elbow Pasta

Another healthy and delicious one pan meal to make your life easier! This meal is nutrient dense and comforting with an unbeatable taste. Completely nut-free and dairy free, egg-free, grain-free, AIP, paleo and Whole30 compliant, this recipe is hard to beat.

8. Easy Dump and Bake General Tso's Chicken

Ingredients:

- ✓ Chicken Breast
- ✓ Broccoli Florets
- ✓ Coconut Sugar
- ✓ AppleCider Vinegar
- ✓ Nomato Sauce
- ✓ Coconut Aminos
- ✓ Fresh and Ground Ginger
- ✓ Crushed Garlic
- ✓ Salt

If you love Chinese takeout, this is a great recipe for you. Extremely fast to assemble and cook, this casserole dish makes a no-fuss, healthy and fresh weeknight meal.

9. AIP Tacos

Ingredients:

- ✓ Pork Lard

- ✓ Onion
- ✓ Ground Beef
- ✓ Carrot
- ✓ Black Olives
- ✓ Avocados
- ✓ Red Onion
- ✓ Lime

Sometimes tacos are difficult to eat on the AIP diet due to various restrictions in toppings and the meat, but we found the perfect recipe to solve all those problems. Quick and easy, everyone loves a good taco.

10. Pork Tenderloin with Blueberry Sauce

Ingredients:

- ✓ Pork Tenderloin
- ✓ Citrus Juice
- ✓ Olive Oil
- ✓ Dried Rosemary
- ✓ Garlic Powder

✓ Ginger Powder

✓ Sea Salt

One of our favorite meals on this list because of the tender, juicy, and flavorful bite of food this dish has to offer. The combination of baked pork tenderloin with a rich decadent blueberry sauce makes for an easy but special dinner.

11. One Pan Apple and Cinnamon Chicken with Bacon

Ingredients:

✓ Chicken Thighs

✓ Bacon Slices

✓ Apples

✓ Cinnamon, Ginger, Cardamom

✓ Rosemary

✓ Sage Leaves

✓ Sea Salt

This dish may sound like the perfect fall meal, and it is, but it's perfect year round too. Warm, comforting, and packed with flavor this is another favorite recipe of ours on the list. With simple ingredients full of nutrients, I'd be eating this meal on a weekly basis.

12. Orange Chicken with Rice

Ingredients:

- ✓ Organic, Pasture-Raised Chicken Breasts
- ✓ Arrowroot Flour
- ✓ Dry seasonings
- ✓ Broccoli Rice
- ✓ Scallions
- ✓ Olive Oil

It's kinda like fast, hot, savory takeout… but better. This homemade orange chicken dish is healthy, organic, and of course AIP friendly. Fast food is pretty much a no-no when it comes to following this diet, so why not make an even better version of this at home?

13. Pulled Pork Stuffed Squash

Ingredients:

- ✓ Squash
- ✓ Pulled Pork
- ✓ Avocado

One of the easiest recipes to make, this recipe is perfect when you're having a super busy day and don't want to put a lot of time or energy into your dinner. And I'll be the first to say, this pulled pork squash does not disappoint.

14. Simple Salmon Cakes

Ingredients:

- ✓ Wild Salmon
- ✓ Carrots
- ✓ Green Onions
- ✓ Lemon
- ✓ Coconut Flour
- ✓ Garlic Powder

✓ Fresh Dill

Salmon is one of the best proteins you can eat while on the AIP diet. These salmon cakes are not only simple to make, but they're more than delicious. Made with carrots instead of egg, these are a healthy and versatile meal that can be eaten at any time of day.

15. Roasted Garlic and Cauliflower Soup

Ingredients:

✓ Cauliflower

✓ Sweet Potato

✓ Garlic

✓ Yellow Onion

✓ Ghee

✓ Olive Oil

✓ Turmeric

✓ Sea Salt

✓ Chicken Broth

This list would not be complete without some soup, and this is as delicious as it gets. This dish offers an incredible depth of flavor and healthy ingredients that will leave you feeling on cloud.

16. Green Banana Fries

Ingredients:

- ✓ Green Bananas
- ✓ Olive Oil
- ✓ Sea Salt

Although this may not necessarily be a full blown meal, green banana fries are one of the best AIP diet snacks. While sweet potato fries are delicious it's hard to get them as crispy as regular fries. That's where these green banana fries come into the picture. Crispy and delicious, you'll hardly know they're not real potatoes.

17. Old Fashioned Original Beef Jerky

Ingredients:

- ✓ Beef
- ✓ Water
- ✓ Seasoning

Now, stay with us for a second. We know Beef Jerky isn't necessarily a recipe; however, it is one of the best snacks out there for the AIP diet. From its healthy ingredients to its simplicity and ease, you can snack on this or use it as a meal replacement. Either way, you thank us later.

18. Meatballs over Spaghetti Squash

Ingredients:

- ✓ Spaghetti Squash
- ✓ Extra Virgin Olive Oil
- ✓ Sea Salt

Made with only 3 ingredients and cooked under an hour, we absolutely love this recipe. Squash is filled with all sorts of nutrients that you should be looking for while following the AIP diet. Quick and easy to prepare, throw some meatballs over your spaghetti squash and have yourself an appetizer or a full blown dinner.

19. Turmeric Zucchini Soup

Ingredients:

- ✓ Coconut Oil
- ✓ Onion
- ✓ Seal Salt
- ✓ Zucchini
- ✓ Garlic
- ✓ Curry Powder
- ✓ Turmeric Powder
- ✓ Vegetable Stock
- ✓ Coconut Milk
- ✓ Fish Sauce
- ✓ Lime Juice
- ✓ Cilantro

Turmeric is an anti-inflammatory spice that also has an incredible taste to it. Combining that with creamy coconut milk, this zucchini soup is healing and nutritious. Light and satisfying, this soup is also paleo, vegan, AIP compliant, and gluten-free. Perfect for anyone with digestive or gut-health problems.

20. Sweet Potato Breakfast Hash

Ingredients:

- ✓ Onion
- ✓ Garlic Cloves
- ✓ Sweet Potatoes
- ✓ Broccoli
- ✓ Apples
- ✓ Salt
- ✓ Coconut Oil
- ✓ Extra Virgin Olive Oil

Perfect for breakfast or dinner, this sweet potato hash is just as delicious as it is easy. You can even easily take this on the go when you're having a busy day or weekend. Customize this recipe by adding any of your favorite vegetables, or even throw in some apples for a unique flavor combination.

21. Crispy AIP Waffles

Ingredients:

- ✓ Tapioca Starch
- ✓ Coconut Flour
- ✓ Avocado Oil
- ✓ Coconut Milk

Easy and quick to make, you'll wish you found this recipe sooner. Although these waffles are not thick and fluffy like traditional waffles, they help give you that sense of eating a normal breakfast again. Plus, they're still delicious.

22. Tuna Heart of Palm Pasta

Ingredients:

- ✓ Hearts of Palm Pasta
- ✓ Wild Canned Tuna
- ✓ Lemon Zest and Juice

- ✓ Extra-Virgin Olive Oil
- ✓ Garlic

We know what you're thinking... pasta? On the AIP diet? Trust us. This pasta is made from the heart of palm, a crunchy vegetable harvested from the center of the cabbage palm tree. Throw some garlic, lemon zest, and tuna on top and you've got yourself a delicious and quick meal.

23. 24-hr Slow Cooker Chicken Broth

Ingredients:

- ✓ Cooked Bones
- ✓ Acid
- ✓ Vegetables
- ✓ Herbs
- ✓ Water

The AIP Diet is all about returning back to a healthy gut, and nothing helps that more than chicken broth. Use this as a base in smoothies or in soups, drink it by itself or turn it into a meal. No matter how you decide to consume this, it's guaranteed to be delicious and nutritious.

24. Picadillo with Plantain Rice

Ingredients:

- ✓ Onion
- ✓ Garlic Cloves
- ✓ Dried Oregano
- ✓ Cumin
- ✓ Cilantro Paste
- ✓ Broth
- ✓ Olives
- ✓ Raisins

Extremely easy to make, you really cannot go wrong with this Picadillo. With a Puerto-Rican type style to it, this dish is sure to do your tastebuds a huge favor. Serve with rice or inside things like a lettuce taco, an empanada, freeze it for later.

25. Stuffed Sweet Potato Skins

Ingredients:

- ✓ Sweet Potatoes
- ✓ Avocado Oil
- ✓ Fine Sea Salt
- ✓ Bacon
- ✓ Mushrooms
- ✓ Red Onion
- ✓ Avocado
- ✓ Scallions
- ✓ Chopped Cilantro
- ✓ Coconut Milk
- ✓ Lemon Juice

One of our favorite recipes on the list, these stuffed sweet potato skins are nutritious, healthy, and fun to eat and share with others. This is an upgrade to those unhealthy regular potato skins we are all guilty to enjoy. Eat these as a snack or as a meal– either way you're going to be more than satisfied.

10 Of The Best Easy Autoimmune Protocol Recipes

These are 10 of the best easy recipes for when following the AIP diet! They're made with easy to find ingredients and many can be made in one pan. The autoimmune protocol can be challenging, especially if you're in the throws of an autoimmune flare. The last thing you want to do is try to decipher recipes that are just too labor intensive if you're not feeling your best.

Though I feel like baked goods and more involved recipes have their place in the AIP when you're really just looking for a special meal or a treat, there is so much opportunity to have meals that are both easy and delicious! These recipes are all easy to make with easy to find ingredients like ground beef, chicken breast, vegetables, and simple staples like coconut aminos, arrowroot starch, cooking fats, and seasonings.

1. Lemon Asparagus Chicken Skillet

This lemon asparagus chicken skillet is a one-pan meal that's made with chicken breast (or thigh), asparagus, chicken broth, coconut aminos, lemon, garlic, and arrowroot starch to thicken the sauce.

2. Egg Roll In A Bowl

Egg roll in a bowl is a simple and flavorful meal that you can make with coleslaw mix, onion, ground pork (or chicken), and coconut aminos. This recipe also uses a ginger cream sauce, but you can leave it off if you'd rather keep it simple.

3. Sweet Potato Chicken Poppers

These sweet potato chicken poppers are one of my most popular recipes! They're made with ground chicken (or turkey), sweet potato that you can rice in the food processor, coconut oil and flour, and some seasonings. I have several other versions like these Mexican Chicken Poppers and Breakfast Sausage Chicken Poppers.

4. One Pan Chicken Pesto

This one-pan chicken pesto is a personal favorite of mine! It's made with an easy homemade pesto made from basil, arugula, olive oil, and lemon, along with chicken and easy to find vegetables.

5. Unstuffed Cabbage Roll

I made this unstuffed cabbage roll recipe after wanting to take a shortcut from actually rolling cabbage rolls! It's made with homemade nomato sauce, onion, cauliflower rice, cabbage, and ground beef.

6. Ground Beef Stir Fry

It doesn't get much easier than this ground beef stir fry. All you need is ground beef, veggies, and coconut aminos for an easy one-pan meal. You can easily mix up the veggies to accommodate whatever you have on hand, and even use other ingredients like ground turkey.

7. Chicken Marsala

This chicken marsala is a simple one-pan meal that actually doesn't use wine, but still has all of the flavors you love of chicken marsala. The main ingredients are chicken breast, mushroom, arrowroot starch, chicken broth, and sherry vinegar (or balsamic vinegar).

8. Spinach Avocado Chicken Burgers

These Spinach Avocado Chicken Burgers are another one of those really easy recipes that I love to make in a pinch! The main ingredients are chicken, spinach, and avocado plus some seasonings. You can easily omit the avocado mayo if you want to keep it simple.

9. Taco Skillet Dinner

This taco skillet is made in one pan with ground beef, onion, garlic, cauliflower rice, avocado, kale, cilantro, and green onion as the main ingredient. Leave out the tomato to keep it AIP.

10. Avocado Tuna Salad

This avocado tuna salad is the ultimate easy meal! All you really need is tuna, avocado, lemon juice, red onion, celery, apple and green onion for a simple lunch.

CONCLUSION

The AIP Diet consists of two phases: the elimination phase and the reintroduction phase. The elimination phase removes potentially harmful foods, and the reintroduction phase slowly reintroduces foods into the diet. The AIP Diet is an anti-inflammatory elimination diet designed to help reduce symptoms associated with autoimmune disorders.

It's composed of two separate phases designed to help you identify and conclusively avoid foods that may trigger inflammation and disease-specific symptoms. While this can be a restrictive diet, you will find various foods to incorporate into your diet within the parameters. The AIP lifestyle may be challenging, especially when you're in the midst of an autoimmune flare.

The last thing you'll want to do is spend your time and energy trying to find recipes you can manage. But don't forget, however difficult things may get on your elimination diet, there are always options for you to explore. Take our Old Fashioned Original Beef Jerky for example. It's quick, easy, nutritious, and AIP diet compliant. Plus, there's always more where that came from. Good luck on your journey!

www.ingramcontent.com/pod-product-compliance
Lightning Source LLC
Chambersburg PA
CBHW061254250726

48653CB00002B/649